EASY SALAD RECIPES

MOUTH-WATERING SALADS TO BOOST YOUR ENERGY

JOHN MCDONALD

Table of Contents

Spanish Salad 7

Avocado salad 9

Waldorf salad 11

Fruit Salad 13

Greek salad with Rice 14

Mango Salsa Salad 16

Red Bean Salad 17

Dill and Butter Squash Salad 19

Fresh cucumber yogurt salad 20

Easy Macaroni Salad 21

Greek Salad with Omelet 23

Bacon and Pea Salad 25

Simple Yellow Salad 26

Citrus and Basil Salad 27

Simple Pretzel Salad 29

Butternut Squash Salad 30

Tomato, Radish and Cucumber Salad 31

Fresh Tomato and Avocado Salad with Dijon Mustard 33

Simple Jicama Salad 34

Fresh Radish and Dill Salad 35

Green Bean and Cabbage Salad 36

Lemony Tangy Cucumber Salad 38

Green Pea Salad with Egg 39

Cherry Tomato and Bacon salad 41

Fresh and Easy Chickpea Salad 42

Hardboiled Egg Salad 43

Tasty Pasta Salad.. 44

Mushroom and Baby Corn Salad with couscous................................. 46

Carrot Salad with Ginger and Lemon 47

Jicama and Water Melon Salad... 48

Fresh Beet Salad... 50

Summer Fresh Cucumber and Watermelon Salad............................. 51

Tasty Onion and Celery Salad.. 52

Spinach and Red Onion Salad 53

Watermelon Topped with Mozzarella 54

Tasty Low-Carb Bacon Salad 55

Fresh Carrot and Cucumber Salad 57

Morning fresh Jicama and Mango salad 58

Healthy and Fresh Tuna Salad... 59

Simple Green Beans, Celery and Olive Salad 61

Spinach Salad with Fresh Mint and Avocado.................................. 62

Fresh Sugar Snaps with Mozzarella... 63

Tuna Salad with Eggs and Apples... 64

Beet and Walnut with Prunes 65

Broccoli florets with Onions and pine nuts.................................... 66

Tofu salad over baby spinach.. 67

Asparagus salad with tasty bacons 69

Easy crabmeat salad... 71

Strawberry and onions tossed in red wine 73

Bulgur with pea nuts and scallions 74

Cornbread crumbs with Tofu salad 76

Tasty bacons with greens 78

Chili salmon salad 80

Avocado and grapefruit salad 81

Quinoa with pine nuts 83

Roasted potato salad with curry powder 84

Mushroom salad with bulgur and quinoa 85

Lemony and Gingery Radish salad 86

Fresh berries and Mango salad 87

Simple Bread and feta salad 88

Smoky trout salad with Julienned Apples 90

Fava with tomatoes and cucumber salad 92

Tasty salad with stale bread 94

Marinated grated salad 96

Cranberry and walnut salad with blue cheese 98

Garlic shrimp salad with peas 99

Fresh Kidney bean salad 101

Tortilla and tomato salad 103

Red Cabbage and carrot salad 105

Strawberry and pear salad with blue cheese 107

Spanish Salad

Ingredients

2 Chopped scallions

2 Pimientos

1 Fresh romaine

6 Olives

1 tsp. Paprika

2 Cloves of garlic

Drizzle of Balsamic vinegar

4 Blanched almonds

2 Bread slices

Pinch of salt to taste

Method

Firstly, preheat the oven. Then grease the grill a bit. Chop the scallions very finely. Now put them in the preheated oven. After they are ready, take them in a mixing bowl and add the fresh romaine, pimientos, olives, and almonds to the bowl. Toss well. Now, add the Balsamic vinegar and sprinkle paprika and salt to taste. Rub the grilled bread slices with garlic and crumble them in the bowl. Toss well.

Enjoy!

Avocado salad

Ingredients

2 fresh avocados

1 freshly chopped sweet onion

1 Finely chopped bell pepper, green

Fresh cilantro, chopped

Juice of 1/2 lemon

Salt to taste

Freshly ground black pepper to sprinkle

Method

Take all the fresh ingredients. Wash them. Now take a mixing salad bowl.

Now add the peeled, pitted and well diced avocado, chopped sweet onion,

chopped green bell pepper, and freshly chopped cilantro. Then drizzle fresh

lime juice of about half a lemon. Then for seasoning sprinkle salt to taste and freshly ground black pepper. Then toss them very well and serve them fresh and delicious.

Enjoy!

Waldorf salad

Ingredients

1/2 cup of mayonnaise

¼ cup Fresh sour cream

¼ cup Chives

1 bunch Fresh parsley, chopped

1 tsp. Lemon zest

Fresh juice of 1/2 a lime

1 tsp. Celery

8 Walnuts

Sugar to taste

Freshly ground black pepper to sprinkle

Method

Take a bowl and pour the mayonnaise and whisk it with fresh sour cream.

Now add the chives, freshly chopped parsley and lemon zest. Mix them well.

Drizzle the fresh lime juice and sprinkle sugar according to your desire and

pepper for seasoning. Toss with chopped celery and walnuts.

Enjoy!

Fruit Salad

Ingredients

2 Fresh red apples

1 cup Cranberries

2-3 stalks of celery

½ cup Chopped walnuts

1 nectarine

Fresh yogurt, according to taste

Method

Take the fresh red apples and chop them well. Chop the walnuts and celery as well. Now take a large mixing salad bowl. Now add the pieces of red apple, Cranberries, Dried or fresh , nectarine, chopped walnuts and chopped fresh celery. Toss well. Now pour the fresh yogurt into the bowl and mix well. Refrigerate the salad for about 3 hours. Serve chilled.

Enjoy!

Greek salad with Rice

Ingredients

½ cup extra virgin olive oil

2 cup cooked rice

1 Fresh cucumber

2 fresh tomatoes

1 bunch fresh parsley

1 bunch mint

1 tsp. dried dill

½ cup Feta cheese

½ cup chopped scallions

Hot sauce, to taste

Salt, to taste

2 tbsp. lemon juice

Lemon zest, to taste

Method

Take a bowl, and whisk extra virgin olive oil, fresh lemon juice and salt to taste. Chop fresh cucumbers and tomatoes. Add them to the olive oil and lemon juice mix and toss to coat. Now add chopped parsley, dried dill, scallions, fresh mint and lemon zest of half a lemon and mix well. Now add in the cooked rice and mix gently to make sure the rice doesn't break up. Top it up with hot sauce and feta cheese. Serve immediately.

Enjoy!

Mango Salsa Salad

Ingredients

1 chopped mango

1 Chopped green onion

3 tbsp. freshly chopped cilantro

3 tbsp. of lemon juice

1 Chopped red bell paper

1 Fine chopped fresh jalapeno pepper

Method

Wash the mango, peel and chop it .Take a mixing bowl and add the mangos, red bell pepper, chopped green onion, freshly chopped cilantro and finely chopped jalapeno pepper. Mix them well. Cover the bowl and allow the mixture to soak in the juices for 30-40 minutes. Place this salsa out in a serving dish and serve it with chips or with fish.

Enjoy!

Red Bean Salad

Ingredients

15 ounces of kidney beans

1 Chopped bell pepper

1 cup Feta cheese

Drizzle of olive oil

1 Minced clove of garlic

1 head Chopped cabbage

1 tsp. Fresh parsley, Chopped

Drizzle of olive oil

Drizzle of fresh lemon juice

Method

First, take the canned kidney beans and rinse well for a few minutes. In a large salad mixing bowl, add the kidney beans, chopped cabbage, onions, bell pepper and minced clove of garlic. Toss together. Then add the parsley,

lemon juice and drizzle olive oil and mix until coated. Top it with feta

cheese. Refrigerate for few hours and serve chilled.

Enjoy!

Dill and Butter Squash Salad

Ingredients

1 fresh sliced zucchini

2 fresh yellow squash

2-3 tsp. of dried dill weed

1 tbsp. Lemon juice

Salt to taste

Pepper

2 tsp. Butter

Method

Wash and chop the zucchini and squash. Heat butter in a pan and sauté the vegetables on low-medium heat for 10-15 minutes. Season the vegetables with a pinch of salt and pepper and dried dill weed. Then sauté for some more time and add the lemon juice. Refrigerate overnight and serve chilled.

Enjoy!

Fresh cucumber yogurt salad

Ingredients

1 cup Plain yogurt

3-4 English cucumbers

Salt

Pepper

1 tsp. Dried dill weed

1 finely chopped shallot

1 clove of garlic minced

Method

Wash the English cucumbers, peel and chop them. Chop the shallot finely. Now take a mixing bowl and add the chopped cucumbers, shallot, yogurt and garlic and mix them thoroughly. Sprinkle salt, pepper and dried dill weed. Toss the salad well. Refrigerate overnight and serve chilled.

Enjoy!

Easy Macaroni Salad

Ingredients

1 cup cooked macaroni

½ cup mayonnaise

3 tbsp. fresh sour cream

1 tsp. dried mustard

1 stalk celery, sliced

1 red onion, chopped

1 tsp. chopped parsley

Sugar, to taste

Drizzle of cider vinegar

Salt to taste

Freshly ground black pepper for seasoning

Method

Take a bowl and whisk mayonnaise along with the fresh sour cream. Add the dried mustard, drizzle of cider vinegar, sugar, salt and freshly ground black pepper to taste. Mix well. Toss in the cooked macaroni and freshly sliced onion, parsley and celery and mix well. Serve immediately.

Enjoy!

Greek Salad with Omelet

Ingredients

5 eggs

1 tbsp. olive oil

½ red onion

2 tomatoes, cut into chunks

5-6 Black olives

1 tsp. chopped parsley

½ cup crumbled feta cheese

Salt and pepper

Method

Take a large bowl and whisk the eggs in it with salt, pepper and chopped parsley. Heat the olive oil in a non-stick pan and fry the red onions for few minutes, until tender. Add tomatoes and olives to the pan and cook for a few minutes. Now, pour the whisked egg into it and cook until done. Scatter the feta cheese on the top and place the pan on the pre-heated grill for 6 minutes. Now, cut the puffed and golden omelet into wedges and serve it.

Enjoy!

Bacon and Pea Salad

Ingredients

4 Slices of bacon

1/4 cup water

2 Fresh onions, finely chopped

1 pack of frozen green peas

A drizzle of Ranch dressing

1/2 cup of cheddar cheese, shredded

Method

Brown the bacon in a pan and crumble when cooked. Keep aside. Boil the pack of green peas in a pot and drain. Cool them. Now take a mixing bowl and combine the crumbled bacon, green peas, onion, ranch dressing and shredded cheddar. Toss them all well and then put in refrigerator for an hour. Serve chilled.

Enjoy!

Simple Yellow Salad

Ingredients

1 cob of Yellow corn

Drizzle of extra virgin olive oil

1 Fresh yellow squash

3 Fresh yellow grape tomatoes

3-4 Fresh basil leaves

Pinch of salt to taste

Freshly ground black pepper to sprinkle

Method

Firstly, cut the kernels off the corn. Cut the fresh yellow squash and fresh yellow grape tomatoes into slices. Now take a skillet and drizzle some olive oil and sauté the corn and squash until tender. In a bowl, add all the ingredients and season to taste. Toss and serve.

Enjoy!

Citrus and Basil Salad

Ingredients

Extra virgin olive oil

2 Oranges, juiced

1 Fresh lemon juice

1 Lemon zest

1 tbsp. of honey

Drizzle of white wine vinegar

Pinch of salt

2-3 Fresh basil leaves, chopped

Method

Take a large salad mixing bowl and add the extra virgin olive oil, fresh lemon and orange juice and mix well. Then add lemon zest, honey, white wine vinegar, fresh basil leaves and sprinkle some salt over them to taste. Toss well to mix. Then put in the refrigerator to chill and serve.

Enjoy!

Simple Pretzel Salad

Ingredients

1 Pack of pretzels

Salt to sprinkle

2/3 cup Peanut oil

Garlic and herb salad dressing, you can use salad dressing of your own choice , according to taste

Method

Take a large mixing bag. Now add the pretzels, peanut oil, the garlic and herb salad dressing mixture or any other salad dressing. Sprinkle some salt to season. Now shake the bag well so that the pretzels are uniformly coated. Serve it immediately.

Enjoy!

Butternut Squash Salad

Ingredients

2 boxes of Butternut squash, Cubed

Drizzle of Extra virgin olive oil

Pinch of salt to taste

Freshly ground black pepper for seasoning

Method

Take about 2 boxes of butternut squash, wash and cube them well. Now, preheat the oven to about 400 degrees F. Take the butternut squash in a bowl, drizzle some extra virgin olive oil and sprinkle a pinch of salt and freshly ground black pepper on them. Toss them well so that all the cubes get uniformly coated. Roast butternut till they soften and top caramelizes. Serve.

Enjoy!

Tomato, Radish and Cucumber Salad

Ingredients

2-3 large tomatoes

1-2 cucumbers

2 radishes, thinly sliced

2 red and orange bell peppers

1 bunch green onions, finely chopped

Drizzle of canola oil

Drizzle of White vinegar

Salt to sprinkle

Pepper to taste

Method

Wash all the vegetables, chop them finely and place in a bowl. Drizzle some canola oil and white vinegar. Toss them well so that all the vegetables get evenly coated. Now sprinkle some salt and freshly ground black pepper and toss again. Serve this fresh salad immediately with bread or chips or with any meal.

Enjoy!

Fresh Tomato and Avocado Salad with Dijon Mustard

Ingredients

2 fresh tomatoes

1 Avocado

1 tsp. of Dijon Mustard

Balsamic vinegar, to taste

Freshly ground black pepper

Little drizzle of extra virgin olive oil

Method

Cut the tomatoes into wedges and peel the avocado, pit and slice it. Take a bowl and mix together the Dijon mustard, a drizzle olive oil, balsamic vinegar to taste and some black pepper. Take a big serving plate and arrange the slices of tomatoes and avocados in it. Now drizzle the dressing that you have prepared over them. Serve this salad immediately.

Enjoy!

Simple Jicama Salad

Ingredients

1 jicama, also known as yam bean

Salt to taste

Drizzle of fresh lime juice

Sprinkle of Chili powder

Method

Peel a jicama and cut into small pieces. Arrange the jicama in a large serving plate. Sprinkle fresh lime juice, salt and chili powder on the pieces of jicama. Serve immediately.

Enjoy!

Fresh Radish and Dill Salad

Ingredients

1 fresh Radish

1½ tsp. of finely chopped dill

3 tsp. white vinegar

Canola oil to drizzle

Pinch of salt

Black pepper, ground

Method

Peel and slice the radish finely. Take the slices in a bowl and add a pinch of salt. Toss well. Let it sit for about 10-12 minutes. Then pour some white vinegar, add the chopped dill, drizzle canola oil and sprinkle pepper. Mix well and serve the dish immediately.

Enjoy!

Green Bean and Cabbage Salad

Ingredients

12 ounces of fresh green beans

1 cup Feta cheese, You can also use Mozzarella

Drizzle of olive oil

1 clove of garlic minced

1 fresh Cabbage

1 tsp. Fresh parsley, Chopped

Drizzle of olive oil

Drizzle of fresh lemon juice

Method

Wash and drain the green beans. In a large salad mixing bowl, add the green

beans, chopped cabbage, onions, garlic, parsley, lemon juice and drizzle

olive oil. Toss well. Top it with feta cheese. Refrigerate to cool and serve.

Enjoy!

Lemony Tangy Cucumber Salad

Ingredients

2-3 fresh cucumbers, finely sliced

2 tsp. white wine vinegar

3 tsp. celery seeds

Salt t, to taste

Fresh black pepper, to taste

4 tbsp. fresh lemon juice

1 chopped onion

Method

Place the cucumbers in salad mixing bowl. Add the white vinegar, celery seeds, onion, lemon juice and sprinkle some salt and some black pepper. Combine everything thoroughly and then put into the freezer. Serve chilled.

Enjoy!

Green Pea Salad with Egg

Ingredients

2 cans fresh green peas

3-4 eggs

4 tbsp. fresh lemon juice

1 tsp. fresh cilantro, chopped

2 fresh onions, chopped

6 cherry tomatoes, cut in halves

Salt to taste

Garlic powder to taste

Method

Mix together the peas, onions, cherry tomatoes, and fresh cilantro. Now squeeze in fresh lemon juice, add some salt, and garlic powder. Mix well. Boil the eggs to make some hard boiled eggs and cut them into halves and add to the salad bowl. Serve immediately.

Enjoy!

Cherry Tomato and Bacon salad

Ingredients

2 fresh cherry tomatoes, cut them into halves

5 slices of bacons

Freshly ground black pepper to taste

Garlic salt to taste

½ cup crumbled fresh mozzarella or feta cheese

Some fresh basil leaves

Method

Cook the slices of bacon until brown, crumble them and keep them in a bowl. Now in a salad mixing bowl, add the halved cherry tomatoes and fresh basil leaves along with crumbled fresh mozzarella or feta cheese over them. Spread the crumbled bacon. Top up with pepper and garlic salt. Serve immediately.

Enjoy!

Fresh and Easy Chickpea Salad

Ingredients

1 can chickpeas

2 red onions, chopped

2 tomatoes, chopped

2 cucumbers, chopped

1 tsp. chili powder

Some salt

Method

Boil the chickpeas in a pot until tender. Place in a mixing bowl with the tomatoes, red onions and cucumber pieces. Combine all of them together very well. Season with salt and chili powder and mix well. Serve it immediately.

Enjoy!

Hardboiled Egg Salad

Ingredients

4-5 hardboiled eggs, chopped

1 Avocado

Dijon mustard, to taste

Pinch of garlic salt to taste

Freshly ground black pepper to sprinkle

Method

Take a bowl and add the pieces of eggs, Dijon mustard, avocado and mash them well together. Sprinkle some garlic salt and pepper to season. Mix them well and serve immediately.

Enjoy!

Tasty Pasta Salad

Ingredients

Cooked Pasta½ cup of mayonnaise

3 tbsp. Fresh sour cream

1 tsp. Dried mustard

1 celery stalk, sliced

1 red onion, chopped

1 tsp. parsley, chopped

Sugar to taste

2 tbsp. White or cider vinegar

Salt, to taste

Freshly ground black pepper, to taste

Method

Take a bowl and whisk mayonnaise along with about fresh sour cream. Add in the dried mustard, drizzle of cider or white vinegar, sugar and sprinkle salt and fresh ground black pepper to taste and mix well. Add the cooked pasta and sliced onion, parsley and celery. Toss them well and serve.

Enjoy!

Mushroom and Baby Corn Salad with couscous

Ingredients

1 cup Couscous

5-6 Mushrooms

1 peeled tomato

7-8 Baby corn

Salt

Black or white pepper

Method

Take a pot with water and add the couscous and bring to boil. When the couscous is cooked drain it well. Meanwhile chop the mushrooms and take in a bowl. Add tomatoes, and baby corn to the mushrooms and microwave for 2 to 3 minutes. Now mix these with the cooked couscous. Mix them well and sprinkle salt and black or white pepper. Serve immediately.

Enjoy!

Carrot Salad with Ginger and Lemon

Ingredients

2 carrots

2 cloves of garlic, minced

1 tsp. cinnamon powder

1/2 inch piece of ginger, grated finely

Salt, to taste

Black pepper, to taste

Drizzle of oil

Method

Wash, peel and slice the carrots and place on a plate. In a bowl, add the grated ginger, garlic, drizzle of oil, cinnamon powder and some pepper and salt. Mix them well. Now spread this mixture with the carrots. Serve immediately.

Enjoy!

Jicama and Water Melon Salad

Ingredients

1 Jicama

1 Watermelon

3 tbsp. fresh lime juice

Lemon zest

2 tsp. Honey

1 tbsp. fresh mint leaves, chopped

Salt and pepper to taste

Method

Cut the jicama into slices and the watermelon into cubes. Place the jicama and water melon in a bowl. Add in the lemon juice, lemon zest, honey and mint. Toss them together so that jicama and watermelons get coated uniformly. Taste and season accordingly. Now refrigerate the salad for about 2 hours and then serve to all.

Enjoy!

Fresh Beet Salad

Ingredients

1 fresh beets, roasted

1tsp. dried mustard powder

Salt

2 onions, chopped

1½ tbsp. poppy seeds

Sugar, to taste

1½ tsp. vegetable oil

½ cup crumbled Feta cheese

Method

Combine all the ingredients in a bowl and toss well till all the ingredients are mixed properly. Serve immediately.

Enjoy!

Summer Fresh Cucumber and Watermelon Salad

Ingredients

2 fresh cucumbers, sliced

1 fresh watermelon, cubed

Pinch of salt to taste

Drizzle of Balsamic vinegar

1 tsp. Sugar

Method

Combine all the ingredients in a bowl and toss well till all the ingredients are mixed properly. Refrigerate and serve.

Enjoy!

Tasty Onion and Celery Salad

Ingredients

1 stalk celery, chopped

2 onions, diced

2 tbsp. Lemon juice

Drizzle of olive oil

5-6 basil leaves

Pinch of salt

Ground pepper, to taste

Method

Combine all the ingredients in a bowl and toss well till all the ingredients are mixed properly. Refrigerate and serve.

Enjoy!

Spinach and Red Onion Salad

Ingredients

1 bunch fresh baby spinach

2 red onions, finely chopped

3 cucumbers, chopped

Crumble some slice of bacons, if you desire

½ cup Fresh Mozzarella cheese

Oregano, to taste

Method

Combine all the ingredients, except for the cheese, in a bowl and toss well till all the ingredients are mixed properly. Refrigerate and serve topped with the cheese.

Enjoy!

Watermelon Topped with Mozzarella

Ingredients

1 Fresh watermelon

5 to 6 fresh Basil leaves

1 tbsp. balsamic vinegar

1 cup Mozzarella cheese

Oregano for seasoning

Method

Combine all the ingredients in a bowl and toss well till all the ingredients are mixed properly. Taste and season accordingly. Refrigerate and serve.

Enjoy!

Tasty Low-Carb Bacon Salad

Ingredients

½ cup of mayonnaise

1 crushed clove of garlic

½ cup lettuce

Salt

Fresh ground black pepper, to taste

4 tbsp. lime juice

1 tbsp. anchovy paste

5 slices of bacon

Method

First take a frying pan and fry the slices of bacon until they become crispy. Cool them and crumble them. Now in a bowl add mayonnaise, garlic salt and pepper and anchovy paste to it. Mix well to form a dressing. Add the fresh lettuce and toss well to coat. Season to taste. Serve topped with the crumbled bacon.

Enjoy!

Fresh Carrot and Cucumber Salad

Ingredients

2 carrots, sliced and roasted

2 cucumbers, sliced

2 tsp. dried mustard powder

Salt

1½ tbsp. poppy seeds

Sugar, to taste

1 1/2 tsp. vegetable oil

½ cup crumbled Feta cheese or mozzarella cheese

Method

Combine all the ingredients in a bowl and toss well till all the ingredients are mixed properly. Serve immediately.

Enjoy!

Morning fresh Jicama and Mango salad

Ingredients

2 fresh mangoes, cubed

1 fresh Jicama, cubed

6-8 fresh mint leaves

Pinch of salt to taste

Drizzle of Balsamic vinegar

Method

Combine all the ingredients in a bowl and toss well till all the ingredients are mixed properly. Refrigerate and serve.

Enjoy!

Healthy and Fresh Tuna Salad

Ingredients

1 mashed avocado

1 scallion, sliced

1 can of tuna

Lime juice, as required

2 tomatoes, finely chopped

Capers, as per taste

Salt to taste

Pepper to taste

Method

Mash the avocado with a fork. Add lime juice to it till the consistency is smooth. Now fold in the chopped tomatoes, drained tuna, capers and scallion into the mashed avocado. Season with salt and black pepper to taste. Serve this delicious tuna salad with chips or with vegetables or on a bed of greens.

Enjoy!

Simple Green Beans, Celery and Olive Salad

Ingredients

1 packet Fresh green beans

1 stalk celery, diced

Lemon juice, as required

Drizzle of olive oil

2 basil leaves

5 Olives

Pinch of salt, to taste

Pepper, to taste

Method

Combine all the ingredients in a bowl and toss well till all the ingredients are mixed properly. Refrigerate and serve.

Enjoy!

Spinach Salad with Fresh Mint and Avocado

Ingredients

1 bunch Fresh baby spinach

Fresh mint, as per taste

2 avocados, sliced

2 red onions, finely chopped

2 cucumbers, chopped

1 cup Mozzarella cheese

Oregano for taste

Method

Combine all the ingredients in a bowl and toss well till all the ingredients are mixed properly. Refrigerate and serve.

Enjoy!

Fresh Sugar Snaps with Mozzarella

Ingredients

1 cup fresh sugar snaps

4 dried cranberries

1 sprig basil leaves

1 sprig mint leaves

Balsamic vinegar, to taste

½ cup fresh Mozzarella cheese

Oregano for seasoning

Method

Combine all the ingredients in a bowl and toss well till all the ingredients are mixed properly. Refrigerate and serve.

Enjoy!

Tuna Salad with Eggs and Apples

Ingredients

1 tuna packed in olive oil

1 fresh green onion, chopped finely

1 apple, sliced

3-4 Hard-boiled eggs

1 tbsp. celery

2 tbsp. cream dressing

Freshly ground black pepper, to taste

Salt, to taste

Method

Combine all the ingredients in a bowl and toss well till all the ingredients are mixed properly. Refrigerate and serve.

Enjoy!

Beet and Walnut with Prunes

Ingredients

2 beets, grated

8 prunes, chopped

2 cloves of garlic, minced

Salt, to taste

1½ tbsp. chopped walnuts

Sugar, as per taste

½ tsp. vegetable oil

½ cup Feta cheese or mozzarella

Method

Combine all the ingredients in a bowl and toss well till all the ingredients are mixed properly. Serve immediately.

Enjoy!

Broccoli florets with Onions and pine nuts

Ingredients

2 cups broccoli florets

1 handful pine nuts

2 red onions, chopped

6-8 mint leaves

2 tsp. balsamic vinegar

½ cup Fresh Mozzarella cheese

Oregano for seasoning

Method

Combine all the ingredients in a bowl and toss well till all the ingredients are mixed properly. Refrigerate and serve chilled.

Enjoy!

Tofu salad over baby spinach

Ingredients

1 Tofu, cubed

1 bunch baby spinach

2-3 pieces of ginger

1/4 cup water

1/2 tsp. Rice wine vinegar

Red chili paste, as per taste

Oil to drizzle

1/2 tsp. soy sauce

Method

Puree the ginger with the water, rice wine vinegar, soy sauce and vegetable oil. Combine the tofu and spinach in a bowl and spoon in the ginger mix onto them.

Enjoy!

Asparagus salad with tasty bacons

Ingredients

1 bunch asparagus, trimmed

1 cup Bacon, crumbled

Drizzle of olive oil

Balsamic vinegar to taste

1 tsp. Soy sauce

Pinch of salt

Ground black pepper

Method

Firstly trim the fresh asparagus and boil them till they are crisp and tender and keep them aside. Now in a small mixing bowl, add some oil, some soy sauce and balsamic vinegar and sprinkle some amount of salt and black ground pepper to taste. Mix them very well. Now in a salad bowl add the asparagus and this dressing and mix. Then add crumbled cooked bacon

pieces and serve immediately.

Enjoy!

Easy crabmeat salad

Ingredients

1 lump of crab meat

1 stalk celery

½ cup mayonnaise

1 tsp. tarragon

2 chives, chopped

1/4 cup fresh sour cream

1 tsp. dried mustard

Fresh lime juice of 1/2 a lemon

Method

First take a deep bowl and mix the lump of crab meat along with the celery

and chives and tarragon. Mix them well. Add the mayonnaise, fresh sour

cream, and dried mustard and drizzle the lime juice. Now mix them all very

thoroughly. Serve immediately.

Enjoy!

Strawberry and onions tossed in red wine

Ingredients

4-5 strawberries, sliced

2 red onions, sliced

½ cup Mayonnaise

¼ of a cup of fresh sour cream

Drizzle of red wine

Some poppy seeds, as per taste

½ cup of white sugar

Method

Combine all the ingredients in a bowl and toss well till all the ingredients are mixed properly. Refrigerate and serve chilled.

Enjoy!

Bulgur with pea nuts and scallions

Ingredients

2 cups cooked bulgur

½ cup peanuts, toasted

2 sprigs scallions

Extra virgin olive oil

2 tomatoes, diced

Fresh parsley

Fresh mint leaves

Salt, to taste

Black pepper, to taste

Method

Combine all the ingredients in a bowl and toss well till all the ingredients are mixed properly. Refrigerate and serve chilled.

Enjoy!

Cornbread crumbs with Tofu salad

Ingredients

1 cup cornbread crumbs

1 Tofu, cubed

2-3 pieces of ginger

Water- as required

2 tsp. white wine vinegar

1 tsp. red chili paste

Oil to drizzle

1 tsp. soy sauce

Method

Take the gingers in a blender and convert into puree by adding some water, white wine vinegar, soy sauce and oil to it. Now once this puree is prepared and spread it over the cornbread crumbs and tofu.

Enjoy!

Tasty bacons with greens

Ingredients

1 bunch trimmed asparagus

1 bunch Baby spinach

1 slice Bacon, crumbled

Drizzle of olive oil

Balsamic vinegar to taste

1 tsp. Soy sauce

Pinch of salt

Ground black pepper

Method

Boil the asparagus till they become tender. In a small mixing bowl, add some oil, some soy sauce and balsamic vinegar and sprinkle some amount of salt and black ground pepper to taste. Mix them very well. Now in a salad bowl add the asparagus, spinach and the dressing and mix. Then add crumbled cooked bacon pieces.

Enjoy!

Chili salmon salad

Ingredients

1 salted salmon, diced

1 stalk celery, chopped

½ cup mayonnaise

2 tomatoes, diced

2 green onions, chopped

½ cup fresh sour cream

2 tsp. red chili paste

Fresh lime juice of 1/2 a lemon

Method

Combine all the ingredients in a bowl and toss well till all the ingredients are mixed properly. Refrigerate and serve chilled.

Enjoy!

Avocado and grapefruit salad

Ingredients

1 avocado

1 grapefruit

2 cloves of garlic

3-4 dried cranberries

½ cup Mayonnaise

¼ cup fresh sour cream

Drizzle of red wine

Some poppy seeds

Pinch of salt and pepper

Method

Combine all the ingredients in a bowl and toss well till all the ingredients are mixed properly. Refrigerate and serve chilled.

Enjoy!

Quinoa with pine nuts

Ingredients

2 cups cooked quinoa

4-5 pine nuts, toasted

Extra virgin olive oil

2 tomatoes, diced

2 tsp. parsley

8-10 mint leaves

Some salt

Pinch of black pepper to taste

Method

Combine all the ingredients in a bowl and toss well till all the ingredients are mixed properly. This salad is best served warm.

Enjoy!

Roasted potato salad with curry powder

Ingredients

2-3 Potatoes, diced and roasted

1 tsp. curry power

½ cup mayonnaise

2 tbsp. vinegar

1 stalk celery, chopped

2 tbsp. chopped cilantro

2 scallions, sliced

Salt and pepper, to taste

Method

Combine all the ingredients in a bowl and toss well till all the ingredients are mixed properly. Serve immediately.

Enjoy!

Mushroom salad with bulgur and quinoa

Ingredients

1 cup cooked Bulgur

1 cup cooked Quinoa

3-4 mushrooms, chopped

2 peeled tomatoes, diced

Salt

Black or white pepper

Method

Place the tomatoes and mushrooms in a microwave safe bowl and heat for 2-3 minutes. Add in rest of the ingredients and mix well. Serve immediately.

Enjoy!

Lemony and Gingery Radish salad

Ingredients

1 radish, boiled and sliced

3 cloves of garlic, minced

1 tsp. cinnamon powder

1 ginger, grated finely

Salt, to taste

Black pepper, to taste

Drizzle of oil

Method

Place the slices of the radish in a plate. Mix the rest of the ingredients to make a dressing. Just before serving pour the dressing over the radish.

Enjoy!

Fresh berries and Mango salad

Ingredients

2 mangoes, cubed

2 strawberries, cut into halves

2 cups blueberries

6-8 mint leaves

Salt to taste

Drizzle of Balsamic vinegar

White sugar, to taste

Method

Combine all the ingredients in a bowl and toss well till all the ingredients are mixed properly. Refrigerate and serve chilled.

Enjoy!

Simple Bread and feta salad

Ingredients

1 loaf of bread, sliced

1 stalk celery, diced

2 tbsp. lemon juice

Drizzle of olive oil

½ cup Feta cheese

2 Fresh basil leaves

8 Olives

Pinch of salt

Pepper, to taste

Method

First take the bread slices and break into pieces. Add the bread, celery, lemon juice, olive oil, olives, basil leaves, and some salt and if you want, then add some pepper. Add in the Feta cheese and refrigerate. Serve chilled.

Enjoy!

Smoky trout salad with Julienned Apples

Ingredients

1 flaked and smoked trout fish

2 tbsp. extra virgin olive oil

1 tsp. horseradish

3 Shallots, minced

1 tsp. Dijon mustard

3 apples, julienned

2 tbsp. vinegar

1 bunch arugula

1 tsp. honey

Pinch of salt

Freshly ground black pepper to taste

Method

Combine all the ingredients in a bowl and toss well till all the ingredients are mixed properly. Serve immediately.

Enjoy!

Fava with tomatoes and cucumber salad

Ingredients

1 can fava beans

2 cucumbers, chopped

2 tomatoes, chopped

1 tbsp. parsley

Fresh juice of 1 lemon

1 tbsp. Oil

2 garlic cloves, minced

Pinch of ground cumin

Pinch of salt

Pinch of pepper

Method

Combine all the ingredients in a bowl and toss well till all the ingredients are mixed properly. Serve immediately.

Enjoy!

Tasty salad with stale bread

Ingredients

1 packet stale bread

2 tbsp. red wine vinegar

2 cloves of garlic, minced

2 red onions, finely chopped

1 stalk celery, chopped

2 tomatoes, diced

2 tbsp. Olive oil

2-3 Basil leaves

Pinch of salt

Pinch of pepper

Method

Marinate the chunks of tomatoes in olive oil and some vinegar for a few hours. Sprinkle some salt and pepper on it and rest for a while. Soak the stale bread in water and then drain them. In a salad mixing bowl, add the soaked bread and marinated tomatoes along with onions, celery and basil. Serve immediately.

Enjoy!

Marinated grated salad

Ingredients

1 head cabbage, grated

2 cucumbers, grated

2 carrots, grated

2 beets, grated

2 onions, sliced

Drizzle of oil

2 tbsp. vinegar

Salt, to taste

Water, as needed

Method

Combine all the ingredients in a bowl and toss well till all the ingredients are mixed properly. Freeze for at least six hours and serve chilled.

Enjoy!

Cranberry and walnut salad with blue cheese

Ingredients

5-6 dried cranberries

2-3 Glazed walnuts

2 oranges, segments cut

Salad dressing, according to taste

Blue cheese, crumbled , for garnish

Some fresh basil leaves

Fresh mint

Method

Combine all the ingredients in a bowl and toss well till all the ingredients are mixed properly. Refrigerate and serve chilled.

Enjoy!

Garlic shrimp salad with peas

Ingredients

5 Small shrimps, boiled

2 tbsp. extra virgin olive oil

2 Minced cloves of garlic

2 Shallots, minced

1 tsp. Dijon mustard

2 tbsp. Vinegar

1 cup Frozen peas, boiled

Pinch of salt

Freshly ground black pepper to sprinkle

Method

Combine all the ingredients in a bowl and toss well till all the ingredients are mixed properly. Serve immediately.

Enjoy!

Fresh Kidney bean salad

Ingredients

1 can of kidney beans

2 cucumbers

2 tomatoes

2 tsp. parsley

Fresh juice of 1 lemon

Oil

2 Cloves of garlic minced

Pinch of ground cumin

Pinch of salt

Pinch of pepper

Method

Now first chop the fresh tomatoes and cucumbers into fine dices. Add the kidney beans to that bowl. Now add the minced cloves of garlic, ground pepper and cumin, pinch of salt to your taste, chopped parsley, drizzle some oil and some fresh lime juice. Toss them very well.

Enjoy!

Tortilla and tomato salad

Ingredients

10 Tortillas, into pieces

2 tbsp. Red wine vinegar

2 Minced cloves of garlic

2 red onions

1 stalk celery

3 Tomatoes

Olive oil

Mozzarella, to garnish

Basil leaves, to garnish

Pinch of salt

Pinch of pepper

Method

Firstly, you have to cut chunks of tomatoes, drizzle some olive oil and some vinegar. Now sprinkle some salt and some pepper. Keep it as it is for few minutes. Now take the tortillas and break them into pieces. In a salad mixing bowl, add tortilla pieces and marinated tomatoes along with onions, celery and basil. Top with mozzarella and serve.

Enjoy!

Red Cabbage and carrot salad

Ingredients

1 head Grated red cabbage

3 Grated carrots

3 Finely sliced onions

Drizzle of oil

2 tbsp. Vinegar

½ cup Mayonnaise

Pinch of sugar

Some milk

Method

First take fresh red cabbage and carrots. Now grate them and put them in a bowl. Now, add some finely sliced onions to this bowl. Now in a separate apparatus, mix the mayonnaise, vinegar, some oil, sugar to taste and some milk. Mix this in the grated vegetables and mix. Keep it in freezer and serve.

Enjoy!

Strawberry and pear salad with blue cheese

Ingredients

10-12 sliced strawberries

10 Glazed walnuts

2 Sliced pears

1 bunch Spinach leaves

Salad dressing, according to taste

Blue cheese, crumbled , for garnish

4-5 basil leaves

Mint

Method

First cut the strawberries and pears into pieces. Now take salad mixing bowl and add some glazed walnuts and fresh spinach leaves. Now spread the salad dressing and mix them thoroughly. Now add the fresh basil leaves and the fresh mints. Then top the dish with blue cheese, crumbled all over the salad. Have I with bread or with anything you wish.

Enjoy!